SIGNS, STAGES AND TREATMENT OF BLADDER CANCER

Detailed knowledge of how to curb bladder cancer.

By

Dr DOUGLAS JASON

Before this document is duplicated or reproduced in any manner, the publisher's consent must be gained.

Therefore, the contents within can neither be stored electronically, transferred, nor kept in a database. Neither in part nor in full can the document be copied, scanned, faxed, or retained without approval from the publisher or creator.

TABLE OF CONTENTS

ABOUT THE AUTHOR

INTRODUCTION

TABLE OF CONTENTS

SIGNS, STAGES AND TREATMENT OF BLADDER CANCER

Detailed knowledge of how to curb bladder cancer.

INTRODUCTION

CHAPTER 1
SIGNIFICANCE OF BLOOD IN URINE.

CHAPTER 2
SYMPTOMS OF BLADDER CHANGES.

CHAPTER 3
SMOKING IS; POSSIBLE CAUSE OF BLADDER CANCER

CHAPTER 4
BLADDER CANCER IS CAUSED BY EXPOSURE TO CERTAIN CHEMICALS

CHAPTER 5
BLADDER CANCER RISK

CHAPTER 6
DIAGNOSIS OF BLADDER CANCER .

CHAPTER 7

CYSTOSCOPY AS A TOOL TO DIAGNOSE BLADDER CANCER.

CHAPTER 8
THE USE OF URINALYSIS AND URINE CYTOLOGY.

CHAPTER 9
USE OF IMAGING INTRAVENOUS PYELOGRAM .

CHAPTER 10
THE USES OF MRI AND CT SCANS

CHAPTER 11

THE FUNCTIONS OF BONE
SCAN IN DIAGNOSING
BLADDER CANCER

CHAPTER 12
Types of Bladder Cancer

CHAPTER 13
TYPES OF TRANSITIONAL
CELL CARCINOMA.

CHAPTER 14
STAGES OF BLADDER
CANCER

CHAPTER 15
Example of Bladder Cancer
Stages using the TNM System

CHAPTER 16
BLADDER CANCER TREATMENT

CHAPTER 17
PARTIAL AND RADICAL CYSTECTOMY.

CHAPTER 18
URINARY DIVERSION AFTER SURGERY.

CHAPTER 19
CHEMOTHERAPY

CHAPTER 20
SIDE EFFECTS OF CHEMOTHERAPY.

CHAPTER 21
IMMUNOTHERAPY AS A
BLADDER CANCER
TREATMENT

CHAPTER 22
USE OF RADIATION TO TREAT
BLADDER CANCER

CHAPTER 23
SURVIVAL RATES AND
PROGNOSIS OF BLADDER
CANCER.

CONCLUSIONS

ABOUT THE AUTHOR

Dr DOUGLAS JASON is a certified dietician who has a strong passion for wellness and a big eagerness to help people all over the world. He uses healthy food, herbs, sauce and other useful tools to help mankind realize its overall goal of optimum health.

INTRODUCTION

The uncontrolled expansion of abnormal bladder or malignant cells on the inner lining of the bladder wall is known as bladder cancer. The majority of bladder cancers are found in their earliest stages when treatment is most effective and the tumor has not migrated outside the bladder. Millions of people worldwide are impacted by the common and potentially fatal condition known as bladder cancer. It is defined by the bladder's aberrant cell development, which can cause several symptoms and consequences. For early detection, efficient management, and better outcomes, it is imperative to be aware of the symptoms, stages, and available bladder cancer treatments. In this post, we'll look at the warning signs and symptoms of bladder cancer, the various stages of the disease's development, and the various treatment options that are available to fight this deadly condition.

CHAPTER 1

SIGNIFICANCE OF BLOOD IN URINE.

Hematuria, or blood in the urine, is one indicator of bladder cancer. Urinary blood is not usually a sign of bladder cancer. Most frequently, other illnesses like trauma, infection, blood abnormalities, kidney issues, exercise, or specific drugs induce hematuria. Gross hematuria, or visible blood in the urine, can be noticed with the naked eye, while microscopic hematuria can only be seen via a urine test. The urine can be discolored, brownish, darker than usual, or, very occasionally, brilliant red.

CHAPTER 2

SYMPTOMS OF BLADDER CHANGES.

Changes in bladder habits, such as the need to urinate more frequently or an urgent urge to urinate without generating urine, can occasionally be brought on by bladder cancer. Pain or burning while urinating without signs of a urinary tract infection is another sign of bladder cancer. These bladder-related symptoms, such as bleeding, are typically brought on by illnesses other than cancer. Bladder cancer can sometimes go unnoticed until it has progressed to a stage where treatment is more challenging.

CHAPTER 3

SMOKING IS; POSSIBLE CAUSE OF BLADDER CANCER

The biggest known risk factor for bladder cancer is smoking, which increases the likelihood of developing the disease by four times compared to nonsmokers. Toxic substances from cigarette smoke are passed into urine by the kidneys after entering the bloodstream through the lungs. This causes a buildup of dangerous substances inside the bladder. According to experts, smoking is responsible for roughly 50% of all bladder malignancies in both men and women.

CHAPTER 4

BLADDER CANCER IS CAUSED BY EXPOSURE TO CERTAIN CHEMICALS

Bladder cancer risk can increase as a result of occupational exposure to specific substances. Metalworkers, hairdressers, and mechanics are among the professions that may expose workers to cancer-causing substances. The dye business uses organic chemicals known as aromatic amines, which are particularly linked to bladder cancer. Follow the suggested safety procedures if you are dealing with dyes, around metal, or making leather, textiles, rubber, or paint. For these workers, smoking ups the danger even further.

CHAPTER 5

BLADDER CANCER RISK

Anyone can develop bladder cancer, although some populations are more susceptible. Bladder cancer is three times as common in men than in women. White persons are twice as likely to get the illness as African Americans and about 90% of instances affect people over the age of 55.

A family history of the disease and prior cancer therapy are two additional risk factors for bladder cancer. Bladder-related birth oddities raise the risk of evolving bladder cancer. The bladder becomes more prone to infection when people are born with a visible or invisible abnormality that connects their bladder with another organ in the belly. This makes the bladder more vulnerable to cellular deviations that can cause cancer. Bladder cancer risk is increased by chronic bladder inflammation (regular bladder infections, bladder stones, and other urinary tract issues that irritate the bladder).

CHAPTER 6

DIAGNOSIS OF BLADDER CANCER .

Even though urine tests may indicate that bladder cancer is present, no one laboratory test can specifically screen for and diagnose the disease. Numerous tests, including urine cytology and assays for tumor marker proteins, may be abnormal if cancer is present.

CHAPTER 7

CYSTOSCOPY AS A TOOL TO DIAGNOSE BLADDER CANCER.

Cystoscopy, a form of endoscopy, is a procedure that enables viewing of the bladder's interior using a small, illuminated tube that houses a camera. If aberrant areas are detected, the device can also take tiny samples (biopsies). The most reliable method for identifying bladder cancer is a tissue biopsy.

CHAPTER 8

THE USE OF URINALYSIS AND URINE CYTOLOGY.

A urine analysis is a very helpful test for both diagnosing and screening for many different diseases and ailments. Any abnormalities in the urine, such as blood, protein, and sugar (glucose), will be found by urinalysis. Urine cytology is the process of examining abnormal cells in urine under a microscope that could be signs of bladder cancer.

CHAPTER 9

USE OF IMAGING INTRAVENOUS PYELOGRAM .

A contrast material (dye) X-ray exam called an intravenous pyelogram is used to visualize the bladder, kidneys, and uterus. The dye used in bladder cancer screening makes the urinary tract's organs more visible, enabling medical professionals to look for probable cancer-specific anomalies.

CHAPTER 10

THE USES OF MRI AND CT SCANS

The detection of tumors and the tracking of cancer metastases, as they spread to different organ systems, are frequently done using MRI and CT images. To look for masses and other abnormalities, a CT scan offers a three-dimensional image of the pelvis, the bladder, and the remainder of the urinary system. Positron emission tomography (PET) and CT images are frequently used to reveal cells with

high metabolic rates. "Hot spots"
of cells with abnormally high
metabolic rates could be signs of
cancer and call for additional
research.

CHAPTER 11

THE FUNCTIONS OF BONE SCAN IN DIAGNOSING BLADDER CANCER

If a tumor is discovered in the bladder, a bone scan may be carried out to check for bone metastases. A modest amount of radioactive material is injected into the veins before the bone scan. Any locations where the skeletal system may have been impacted by the malignancy will be visible on a full body scan.

CHAPTER 12

Types of Bladder Cancer

The particular cell type that develops into cancer is what gives bladder tumors their name. The majority of bladder malignancies are transitional cell carcinomas, so named after the bladder lining cells. Squamous cell carcinoma and adenocarcinoma are two other, less prevalent varieties of bladder cancer.

Converging Cell Carcinoma Transitional cell carcinoma is the name for bladder cancer that develops inside the bladder's deepest tissue layer, the transitional epithelium. When the bladder is full, these cells can expand, and when it is empty, they can contract. The transitional epithelium is where the majority of bladder tumors start.

CHAPTER 13

TYPES OF TRANSITIONAL CELL CARCINOMA.

Low-grade and high-grade transitional cell carcinomas are the two forms. After treatment, low-grade transitional cell carcinoma frequently returns, but it seldom spreads to the bladder's muscle layer or other regions of the body. After treatment, high-grade transitional cell carcinoma frequently recurs and spreads to the lymph nodes, other body areas, and the bladder's muscle layer. Most bladder cancer deaths

are brought on by high-grade
illnesses.

Cancer of the Squamous Cells
Squamous cells are flat, thin cells
that might cause bladder cancer if
they are irritated or infected for an
extended period.

Adenocarcinoma
The bladder's glandular cells give
rise to adenocarcinoma tumors.
An extremely uncommon variety
of bladder cancer is
adenocarcinoma.

CHAPTER 14

STAGES OF BLADDER CANCER

The degree to which cancer has developed or spread is frequently used to identify the stage of the disease. A staging system is a technique for medical practitioners to indicate precisely how far along a malignancy is. The TNM system, which is frequently applied to bladder cancer, stands for the following:

T details the progression of the primary tumor.

N identifies any malignancy that has progressed to the bladder's nearby lymph nodes.
M indicates if the cancer has metastasized (spread) to other organs besides the bladder.

CHAPTER 15

Example of Bladder Cancer Stages using the TNM System

The malignancy is a non-invasive papillary carcinoma and has not spread to the connective tissue or the muscle of the bladder wall. Stage 0a (Ta, N0, M0).

Stage 0is (Tis, N0, M0): Only cancerous cells in the bladder's inner lining tissue.

Stage I (T1, N0, M0): The bladder wall has been infiltrated by the tumor.

Stage II (T2, N0, M0): The bladder wall muscle has been affected by the tumor, which has pierced the inner wall.

Stage III (T3, N0, M0): The tumor has metastasized to the fat surrounding the bladder through the bladder.

Any one of the following is Stage IV: (T4, N0, M0): A tumor has penetrated the bladder wall and entered the abdominal or pelvic wall.

Any T, N1, or M0: The lymph nodes adjacent have become infected by the tumor. Any T, any N, M1: The tumor has metastasized to far-off lymph nodes or organs like the liver, lungs, or bones.

CHAPTER 16

BLADDER CANCER TREATMENT

Transurethral Resection in
Surgery
Transurethral surgery is most
frequently used to treat early-
stage malignancies. The urethra is
used as a passageway for a
device called a resectoscope that
is put into the bladder. To retrieve
a tumor from the bladder, the loop
uses an electrical current to cut or
burn the tumor.

CHAPTER 17

PARTIAL AND RADICAL CYSTECTOMY.

Part of the bladder is removed during a partial cystectomy. This procedure is typically used to treat low-grade tumors that have only affected a small portion of the bladder but have already infiltrated the bladder wall. A radical cystectomy involves the complete removal of the bladder, along with any nearby lymph nodes and any malignant tissue. Other organs, such as the uterus and ovaries in women and the prostate in men, may also be removed if cancer has spread outside of the bladder and into the surrounding tissue.

CHAPTER 18

URINARY DIVERSION AFTER SURGERY.

The surgeon will devise a different system for storing and excreting urine after removing the entire bladder. Urinary diversion is the practice in question. To collect urine, a bag may be put either within or outside the body, depending on desire. When a urostomy bag is worn underneath the clothing and put outside the body, this is referred to as non-continent urinary diversion. In a continent urinary diversion, urine is stored in an internal pouch comprised of intestinal tissue. The placement of an artificial bladder has also proven helpful for some individuals following a recently established surgical method.

CHAPTER 19

CHEMOTHERAPY

In some situations, chemotherapy is administered before surgery to reduce bladder cancer tumors. It can also be administered after surgery to kill any leftover tumor cells. Chemotherapy may be delivered intravenously or administered directly into the bladder (intravesical chemotherapy). Intravesical chemotherapy is beneficial in decreasing the recurrence rate of superficial bladder malignancies on a short-term basis, but not effective against bladder cancer that has already infiltrated the muscle walls. Systemic or intravenous chemotherapy is indicated when the cancer has deeply entered the bladder, lymph nodes, or other organs.

CHAPTER 20

SIDE EFFECTS OF CHEMOTHERAPY.

Patients experience side effects differently. The following are typical side effects of systemic chemotherapy:

nausea and diarrhea
reduced appetite
Hair loss
Sores on the interior of the mouth or in the digestive system
Feeling weary or lacking energy
Increased susceptibility to infection
Simple bleeding or bruises

tingling or numbness in the hands
or feet

CHAPTER 21

IMMUNOTHERAPY AS A BLADDER CANCER TREATMENT

To get the immune system to target both the bacteria and the cancer cells, immunotherapy entails injecting beneficial bacteria through a catheter into the bladder. Only bladder tumors in stages Ta, T1, and CIS (carcinoma in situ) are treated with immunotherapy. This treatment employs a particular kind of bacteria called Bacillus Calmette-Guerin (BCG). After surgery, intravenous BCG therapy can be utilized to reduce the likelihood of tumor recurrence. This therapy is administered once per week. Side effects of immunotherapy may include flu-like symptoms, bladder discomfort, and mild bladder hemorrhage.

CHAPTER 22

USE OF RADIATION TO TREAT BLADDER CANCER

Describe radiation.
The use of painless, invisible, high-energy radiation that can kill both healthy and malignant cells is known as radiation therapy. To kill cancer cells, radiation can be used instead of or in addition to chemotherapy and surgery.

Outside Radiation
A device external to the body emits radiation into the environment. A targeted radiation beam is directed at the tumor by

the equipment. For five to seven weeks, external radiation is normally administered five days each week.

Occupational Radiation

The procedure for internal radiation involves putting a tiny radioactive pellet inside the bladder. Patients must remain in the hospital throughout the treatment till the pellet is taken out.

Radiation Consequences

Additionally, radiation therapy might cause adverse effects like diarrhea, tiredness, nausea, and skin irritation.

CHAPTER 23

SURVIVAL RATES AND PROGNOSIS OF BLADDER CANCER.

Rates of Survival for Bladder Cancer
The stage or degree of cancer's spread when it is discovered determines the survival rates, as it does for the majority of malignancies. When the tumor is confined to the bladder's inner

lining, it is possible to identify about 50% of bladder cancers, and patients who are diagnosed at this early stage of the disease have approximately 100% 5-year survival rates. Lower survival rates are normal for cancers that have gone farther. At five years, ten years, and fifteen years, respectively, the relative survival rates for bladder cancer in all stages are 77%, 70%, and 65%.

The prognosis for Bladder Cancer
The prognosis for people with bladder cancer varies on the cancer's stage at the time of diagnosis. The typical prognosis for patients with metastatic

bladder cancer that has progressed to other organs is 12 to 18 months. Recurrent cancer indicates a more aggressive form and a poor prognosis for long-term survival in bladder cancer patients.

Sex Following Bladder Cancer Therapy

Surgery to treat bladder cancer may harm pelvic nerves, making sex uncomfortable.

Men's Changes

Some men could have problems getting an erection, however, this might get better over time for younger guys. If both the prostate gland and the seminal vesicles were removed during surgery, no sperm could be generated.

Adaptations for Women
In women, a radical cystectomy involves the removal of the uterus, ovaries, and a portion of the vagina. This prevents future pregnancies and ends menstruation permanently. It's possible for women who have surgery for bladder cancer to experience uncomfortable sex and have trouble eliciting orgasms.

CONCLUSIONS

There are no complementary or alternative treatments that have been demonstrated to prevent or treat bladder cancer. Green tea and broccoli sprouts are currently being studied as potential alternative therapies. Any such "therapies" should be discussed with your doctor before beginning. Although there is currently no proven technique to prevent bladder cancer, maintaining a healthy lifestyle is always recommended. Quit smoking and restrict your daily alcohol intake to 1 to 2 drinks. Lots of fruits, vegetables, complete grains, and

lean meats in the right portions
make up a nutritious diet.
Additionally, regular exercise and
checkups can improve your health
and provide you peace of mind.
When dealing with chemicals,
keep yourself protected and avoid
harmful chemical exposures.